ALKALINE COOKBOOK FOR BEGINNERS

Delicious Recipes & 30-Day Detox Meal Plan to Kickstart Your Health Journey

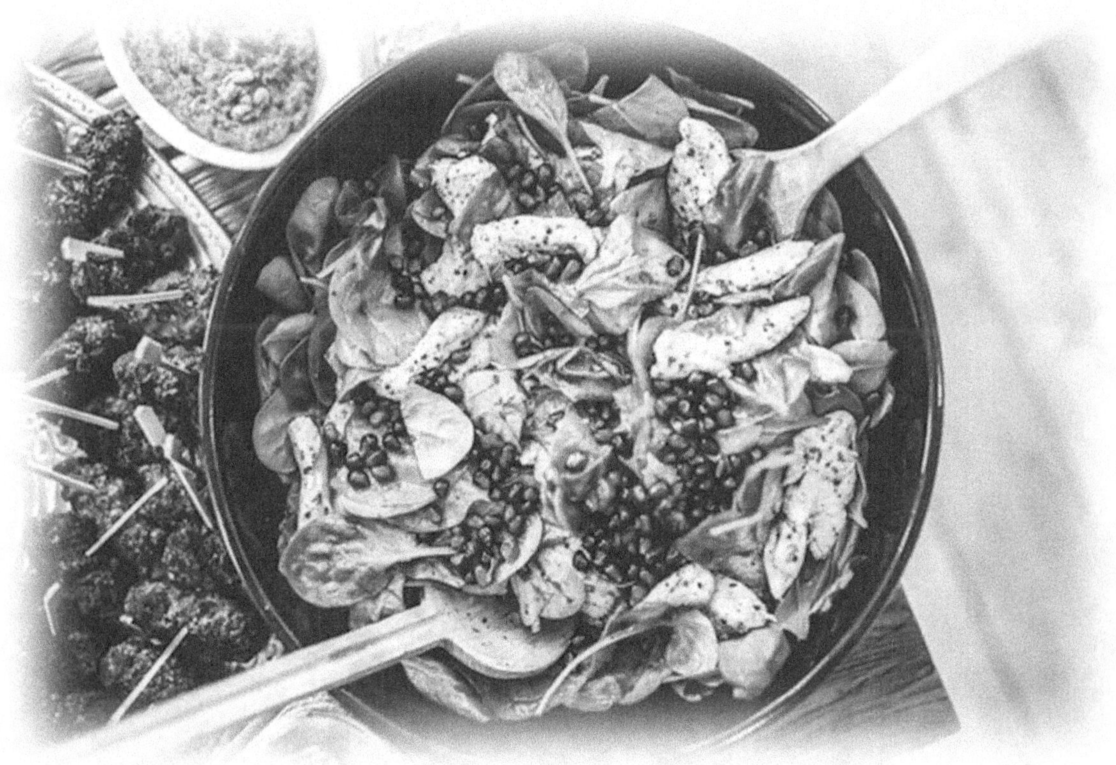

Christiana White

GAIN ACCESS TO MORE BOOKS

DISCLAIMER

The recipes in this cookbook are provided for informational purposes only and are not intended as medical or professional advice. While the author and publisher have made every effort to ensure the accuracy and effectiveness of the recipes, they are not responsible for any adverse effects r consequences resulting from the use of the suggestions herein.

The information in this cookbook should not replace professional advice. Readers are advised to consult a healthcare provider or a culinary professional before making any significant changes to their diet or cooking practices.

Nutritional information is approximate and should be used as a guide only. Variations may occur due to product availability, food preparation, portion size, and other factors.

The author and publisher disclaim any liability in connection with the use of this information. It is the reader's responsibility to determine the value and quality of any recipe or instructions provided for food preparation and to determine the nutritional adequacy of the food to be consumed.

ABOUT THE AUTHOR

When it comes to tasty and nutritious cookbooks that turn wellness into a delightful journey, Christiana White is the author you turn to. She approaches cooking from a new angle and has a passion for creating wholesome food.

Motivated by her own pursuit of health, Christiana's books on Amazon are brimming with delectable recipes that demonstrate that eating healthily can be both simple and enjoyable. Her creative method makes cooking approachable to all skill levels by fusing entire, simple foods with flavors from around the world.

Readers of Christiana's meals gush about the beneficial effects her foods have on their lives outside of the kitchen. Her books are more than just recipes; they're guides for a happier, better way of life, resulting in everything from more energy to a revitalized passion for cooking.

Come along with Christiana to discover how to turn your meals into satisfying and joyful experiences. Discover the delightful intersection of health and flavor by delving into the colourful world of her cookbooks.

TABLE OF CONTENTS.

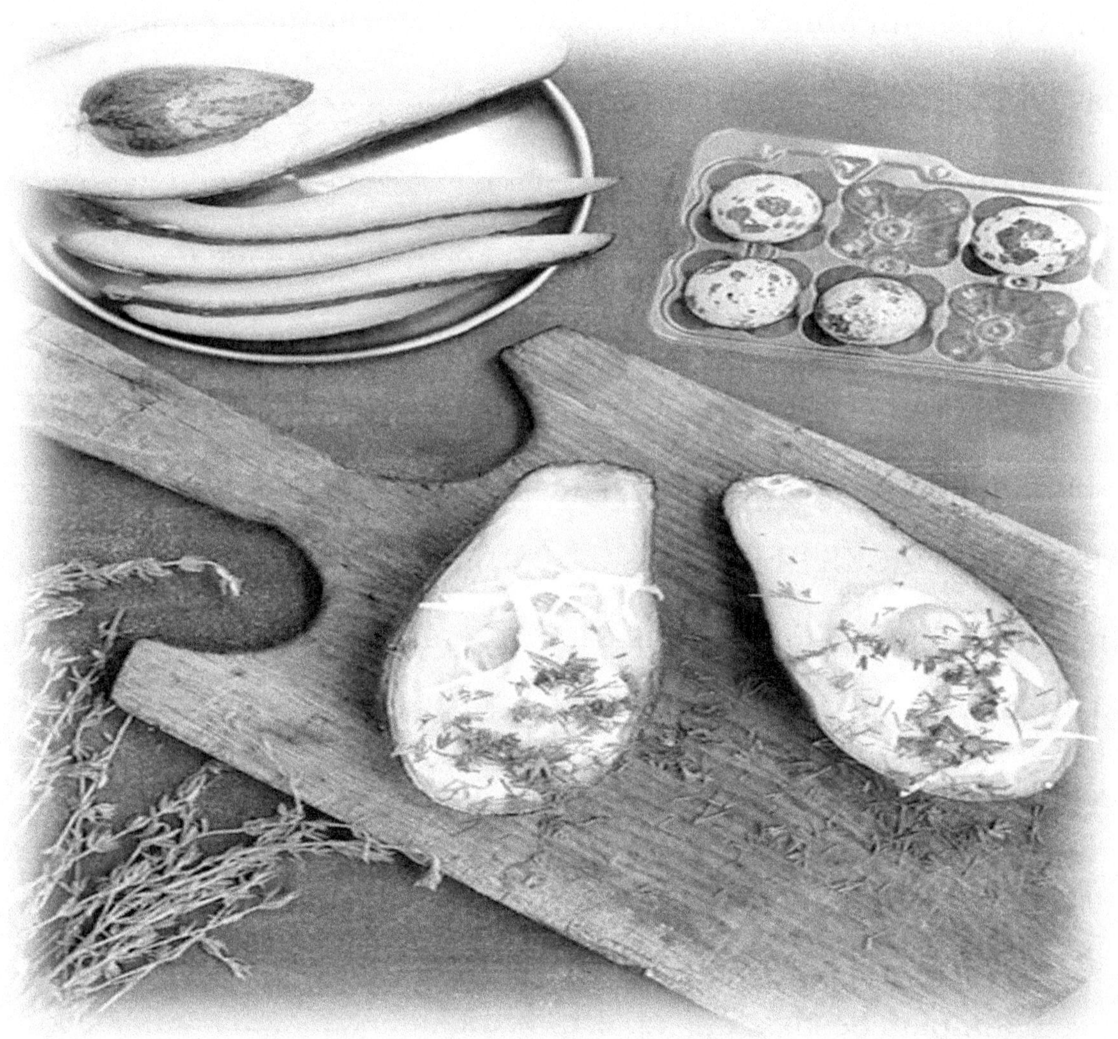

INTRODUCTION

Imagine waking up every morning feeling refreshed, with a nourished body and a clear mind. This is not a pipe dream for individuals who live an alkaline lifestyle. "Alkaline Cookbook for Beginners" is your ticket to better health, one delicious meal at a time.

In these pages, you'll learn the secrets of the alkaline diet, which promotes balance, Vigor, and life. You will learn not just what to eat, but also how to approach food in a new and comprehensive way. This isn't a fad diet; it's a return to the fundamentals of healthy eating for life.

This cookbook is more than just a collection of dishes; it's a full guide to a new you. It includes a 30-day detox plan to reset your system, recommendations for a long and healthy life, and guidelines for navigating potential side effects.

Whether you're a seasoned cook or just beginning in the kitchen, the recipes on these pages are intended to be simple, satisfying, and completely alkaline. From stimulating breakfasts to hearty dinners, each dish represents a step toward better health.

So, are you ready to go on a gastronomic journey that will take you to a healthier, more balanced version of yourself? "Alkaline Cookbook for Beginners" is the companion you have been looking for. Let us begin this transformative journey together.

Welcome to Alkaline Eating

Beginning the journey of alkaline food is like opening the door to a garden of vibrant health and wellness. This portion of your cookbook will be the foundation for learning the fundamentals of an alkaline diet and how it might improve one's life.

Alkaline diet is based on the idea that particular meals can alter the acidity and alkalinity of physiological fluids, such as blood and urine. The diet focuses on eating more alkaline-promoting foods, such as fruits, vegetables, nuts, and seeds, while avoiding acidic foods such as meat, fish, dairy, and processed grains.

Here's what readers may expect to learn from this informative section:

- The Science of Alkalinity: A simple explanation of the body's pH balance and how an alkaline diet promotes this delicate balance.
- Benefits of Alkaline Eating: A comprehensive look at the numerous health benefits linked with an alkaline diet, ranging from enhanced energy to improved digestion and beyond.
- Alkaline Foods to Love: A comprehensive list of alkaline foods that will serve as the foundation for the reader's new dietary habits, along with suggestions for incorporating them into everyday meals.
- Acidic Foods to Limit: Advice on which foods to consume in moderation, allowing readers to make informed decisions without feeling deprived.

- Transitioning to Alkaline Eating: Practical suggestions for gradually transitioning to an alkaline diet while keeping the change sustainable and pleasurable.

The Power of pH Balance

In the realm of health and nutrition, few concepts hold as much significance as the power of pH balance. It is the golden thread that runs through all aspects of the alkaline diet, supporting its philosophy and promising a slew of health advantages. But what exactly is pH balance, and why is it so important?

The term pH stands for "potential of hydrogen" and refers to the concentration of hydrogen ions in a solution. The pH scale spans from 0 to 14, with 7 being neutral. Anything below 7 is acidic, whereas anything above 7 is alkaline. The human body maintains a narrow pH range, with blood pH resting between 7.35 and 7.45. This tiny window is important to the body's overall operation; even minor deviations can have serious consequences for our health.

Why pH Balance is Crucial

Our bodies are continuously seeking for equilibrium, and pH balance is an important element of that. Enzymes, which catalyze practically every metabolic reaction in our cells, require a precise pH level to work properly.

When the body's pH is off, it can cause a slew of health problems, ranging from weariness and inflammation to more serious disorders like osteoporosis and chronic kidney disease.

The Alkaline Diet Connection

The alkaline diet is based on the premise that eating more alkaline-forming foods and less acid-forming foods will assist our bodies maintain healthy pH levels. Most fruits, vegetables, nuts, and seeds are alkaline, whereas meats, dairy, processed foods, and sweets are acidic.

Benefits of an alkaline pH

Adopting an alkaline diet has various health benefits, including:

- Enhanced Bone Health: An alkaline environment helps the body retain bone density and lowers the incidence of osteoporosis.
- Improved Digestion: An alkaline pH promotes good bacteria in the gut, which can help with typical digestive problems.
- Increased Energy and Vitality: Many people report feeling more energized and thinking clearly after following an alkaline diet.
- Detoxification: Keeping the body alkaline can help it discharge toxins more efficiently.
- Weight Management: An alkaline diet can help balance hormones and reduce inflammation, hence promoting weight loss and management.

Maintaining pH balance.

- Monitor Your Diet: Keep a food journal to measure the pH of your meals.
- pH Strips: Check your saliva or urine's pH on a regular basis.
- Stay Hydrated: Drink plenty of alkaline water or water with lemon juice.
- Regular exercise helps to maintain pH equilibrium by lowering acid buildup in the body.

The power of pH balance demonstrates the body's extraordinary ability to control itself. Understanding and harnessing this power through the alkaline diet can help us live a better, more vibrant life. This cookbook contains not only recipes, but also a guide to a healthy and rewarding diet.

How to Use This Cookbook

Welcome to "Alkaline Cookbook for Beginners," your full guide to living an alkaline lifestyle with tasty and nutritious dishes. This cookbook aims to be user-friendly, instructive, and inspiring. Whether you're a beginner in the kitchen or a seasoned cook eager to experiment with the alkaline diet, this book will act as your culinary guide.

Here's how to get the most out of this cookbook.

- Start by reading the introductory parts, which describe the alkaline diet's concept and benefits. Understanding the 'why' behind your dietary choices is equally vital as the 'how.'
- The Table of Contents provides an overview of the book's structure. It is designed to guide you through the fundamentals of alkaline diet before on to more complex concepts and recipes.
- If you are new to the alkaline diet, the 30-Day Detox Plan is an excellent place to begin. It is a step-by-step method for resetting your body and palate.
- Explore the recipes area, which is organized into sections such as Breakfast, Plant-Based, Seafood, Meat, and Snacks. Each category contains a range of dishes to fit your tastes and nutritional needs.

- Make use of the Shopping Plan to stock your kitchen with alkaline-friendly foods. This will make dinner preparation more convenient and fun.
- Use the suggestions and strategies in the book to improve your culinary experience and live a healthy, alkaline lifestyle.
- Feel free to experiment with the recipes. The measurements and ingredients are suggestions; modify them to suit your preferences and dietary requirements.
- Keep track of your favourite recipes and any adjustments you make. This will help you construct your own alkaline diet.
- Use this cookbook as a discussion starter with your friends and family. Share your experiences and favourite recipes to inspire others.
- Use this cookbook as a starting point. Continue to educate yourself on alkaline eating and how it might fit into your lifestyle.

By following these instructions, you'll not only learn how to make tasty alkaline meals, but also how they help you become healthier and more balanced. Enjoy the journey and let the flavors and wisdom contained inside these pages nourish your body and soul.

CHAPTER 1: UNDERSTANDING THE ALKALINE DIET

The alkaline diet is a lifestyle choice that can improve one's health and well-being. This chapter will help you understand the alkaline diet and make informed nutritional selections.

Benefits of Alkaline Living

Adopting an alkaline lifestyle represents a dedication to your health and well-being. It's about making deliberate decisions that support your body's natural state of balance. The advantages of alkaline living are numerous and can result in substantial changes in how you feel, both physically and mentally.

Enhanced Physical Health

- Improved Digestive Function: An alkaline diet supports gut health by stimulating the growth of good bacteria while also lowering inflammation.
- Bone Strength: Alkaline minerals are essential for preserving bone density and avoiding osteoporosis.
- Muscle Efficiency: Maintaining an alkaline state helps to preserve muscle mass as you age, allowing you to remain strong and agile.
- Cardiovascular Health: An alkaline diet can help prevent plaque buildup in blood vessels, hence promoting heart health.

Increased Energy Levels

- Sustained Energy: Alkaline meals can assist to regulate blood sugar levels, delivering continuous energy throughout the day.
- Better Sleep: The minerals in alkaline diets promote peaceful sleep, which is necessary for energy production.

Improved Mental Wellbeing

- Cognitive Function: An alkaline diet promotes brain health, which may improve memory and concentration.
- Mood Stability: The diet can alter neurotransmitter production, potentially improving mood and reducing stress.

Detoxification

- Natural Detox: Alkaline foods aid in the body's natural detoxification processes, allowing it to discharge toxins more efficiently.
- Improved Liver Function: An alkaline diet can help the liver perform its duty as the body's primary detoxification organ.

Weight Management

- Appetite Control: Alkaline foods are generally high in fibre, which can aid in appetite regulation and weight management.
- Metabolic Support: The diet can help increase metabolism, making it simpler to stay at a healthy weight.

Skin Health.

- Clearer Skin: Alkaline living can improve skin clarity and elasticity by improving hydration and nourishment.
- Anti-Aging: Antioxidant-rich alkaline meals can help fight oxidative stress, which is connected to aging.

Prevention of Chronic Disease

- Reduced Inflammation: Many alkaline foods have anti-inflammatory compounds that can help avoid chronic diseases.
- Cancer Risk Reduction: According to some study, eating an alkaline diet may reduce your risk of some types of cancer.

Environmental Impact

- Sustainable Choices: Consuming more plant-based, alkaline foods often results in a lower environmental footprint.

By adopting alkaline principles into your life, you are not only choosing healthy meals; you are also choosing a lifestyle that fosters harmony inside your body and with the world around you.

The benefits of alkaline living extend beyond the plate, providing a comprehensive approach to health that can change your life.

Foods to Embrace and Avoid

Navigating the world of alkaline diet might be intimidating at first, but knowing which foods to embrace and which to avoid is critical for reaching pH balance and reaping the benefits of this lifestyle. Let's break it down into basic, easy-to-follow guidelines:

Alkaline-Forming Foods to Enjoy:

- veggies: A staple of an alkaline diet, veggies are high in important minerals and antioxidants. Fill your plate with leafy greens (kale, spinach, collard greens), cruciferous vegetables (broccoli, cauliflower, Brussels sprouts), root vegetables (sweet potatoes, beets, carrots), and other colorful vegetables such as cucumbers, peppers, and tomatoes.
- Fruits: Although certain fruits are slightly acidic, they provide vital nutrients and fibre. Choose low-sugar fruits such as berries, lemons, limes, avocados, and watermelons.
- Nuts & Seeds: These nutritional powerhouses are high in good fats, protein, and minerals. Almonds, chia seeds, flax seeds, pumpkin seeds, and hemp seeds are all great alternatives.
- Legumes: Black beans, lentils, chickpeas, and other legumes are good sources of plant-based energy and fibre, which helps keep the environment alkaline.
- Herbs and spices: Add flavour to your recipes with herbs like basil, parsley, and cilantro, as well as spices like ginger, turmeric, and cinnamon, all of which have extra health advantages.

- Staying hydrated with alkaline water can help neutralize acids and maintain pH equilibrium.

Limit or avoid the following acid-forming foods:

- Processed foods: These include fast food, sugary cereals, packed snacks, and refined grains. These are frequently heavy in sugar, bad fats, and artificial substances, which add to acidity.
- Refined Sugar: White sugar, high fructose corn syrup, and artificial sweeteners alter pH balance and promote inflammation.
- Animal Products: Meat, poultry, dairy, and eggs are all considered acid-forming. While some people incorporate modest amounts of these items into their alkaline diet, it is recommended to limit them or opt for organic and grass-fed alternatives.
- Grains: Wheat, barley, and other grains are slightly acidic. If you include them, choose whole grains in moderation.
- Alcohol and caffeine: These beverages can upset the body's pH equilibrium and dehydrate it, causing increased acidity.
- Carbonated beverages, such as sodas, should be avoided due to their high acid content.

Neutral foods:

Some foods, such as healthy fats (olive oil, avocado oil, coconut oil) and specific grains (quinoa, millet), are neutral and can be consumed in moderation as part of an alkaline diet.

The 80-20 Rule:

Remember that alkaline eating is about achieving balance more than perfection. Aim to load your plate with 80% alkaline-forming meals and 20% acid-forming or neutral items. This strategy guarantees that you acquire a range of nutrients while maintaining a healthy pH level.

By making thoughtful choices and emphasizing alkaline-forming foods, you may establish a long-term and joyful eating pattern that nourishes your body and promotes health.

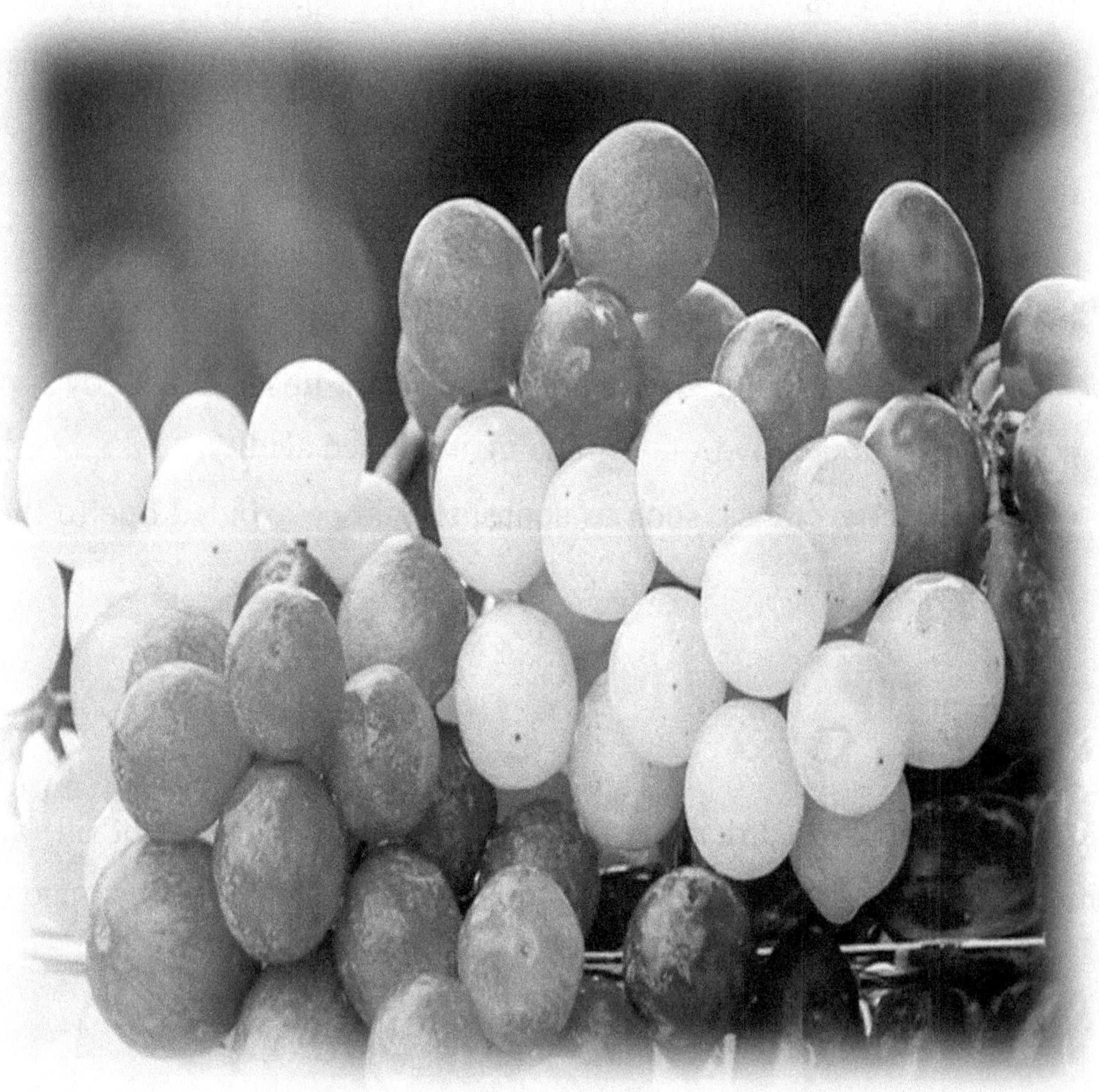

CHAPTER 2: THE 30-DAY DETOX PLAN

Week 1: Kickstarting Alkalinity

Monday

- Breakfast: Alkaline Green Smoothie
- Lunch: Kale and Avocado Salad
- Dinner: Grilled Lemon-Garlic Salmon

Tuesday

- Breakfast: Quinoa Fruit Salad
- Lunch: Quinoa Stuffed Bell Peppers
- Dinner: Herb-Crusted Cod

Wednesday

- Breakfast: Spelt Pancakes
- Lunch: Spicy Chickpea Stew
- Dinner: Grilled Chicken with Herb Salad

Thursday

- Breakfast: Chia Seed Pudding
- Lunch: Butternut Squash Soup
- Dinner: Seafood Quinoa Paella

Friday

- Breakfast: Buckwheat Porridge
- Lunch: Zucchini Noodles with Pesto
- Dinner: Turkey Meatballs in Tomato Sauce

Saturday

- Breakfast: Kamut Flour Waffles
- Lunch: Lentil and Vegetable Curry
- Dinner: Beef Stir-Fry with Alkaline Vegetables

Sunday

- Breakfast: Alkaline Avocado Bowl
- Lunch: Stuffed Portobello Mushrooms
- Dinner: Lamb Chops with Mint Pesto

Snacks (Choose One Daily):

- Almond Butter and Celery Sticks
- Kale Chips
- Cucumber and Hummus Bites
- Coconut Yogurt with Nuts and Seeds

Week 2: Deepening Alkaline Habits

Monday

- Breakfast: Millet and Cinnamon Apple Bowl
- Lunch: Wild Rice and Mushroom Pilaf
- Dinner: Roasted Duck with Orange Glaze

Tuesday

- Breakfast: Amaranth Porridge with Berries
- Lunch: Eggplant and Tomato Bake
- Dinner: Venison Stew with Root Vegetables

Wednesday

- Breakfast: Teff Grain Breakfast Bowl
- Lunch: Sweet Potato and Black Bean Chili
- Dinner: Pork Tenderloin with Apple Compote

Thursday

- Breakfast: Alkaline Green Smoothie
- Lunch: Kale and Avocado Salad
- Dinner: Buffalo Cauliflower Bites

Friday

- Breakfast: Quinoa Fruit Salad
- Lunch: Quinoa Stuffed Bell Peppers
- Dinner: Chicken Avocado Lettuce Wraps

Saturday

- Breakfast: Spelt Pancakes
- Lunch: Spicy Chickpea Stew
- Dinner: Bison Burgers with Alkaline Slaw

Sunday

- Breakfast: Chia Seed Pudding
- Lunch: Butternut Squash Soup
- Dinner: Grilled Lemon-Garlic Salmon

Week 3: Integrating Alkaline Diversity

Monday

- Breakfast: Buckwheat Porridge
- Lunch: Zucchini Noodles with Pesto
- Dinner: Herb-Crusted Cod

Tuesday

- Breakfast: Kamut Flour Waffles
- Lunch: Lentil and Vegetable Curry
- Dinner: Seafood Quinoa Paella

Wednesday

- Breakfast: Alkaline Avocado Bowl
- Lunch: Stuffed Portobello Mushrooms
- Dinner: Alkaline Fish Tacos

Thursday

- Breakfast: Millet and Cinnamon Apple Bowl
- Lunch: Wild Rice and Mushroom Pilaf
- Dinner: Mussels in Tomato Broth

Friday

- Breakfast: Amaranth Porridge with Berries
- Lunch: Eggplant and Tomato Bake
- Dinner: Scallops with Zesty Quinoa

Saturday

- Breakfast: Teff Grain Breakfast Bowl
- Lunch: Sweet Potato and Black Bean Chili
- Dinner: Tuna and Avocado Poke Bowl

Sunday

- Breakfast: Alkaline Green Smoothie
- Lunch: Kale and Avocado Salad
- Dinner: Sardine and Spinach Salad

Week 4: Establishing Alkaline Mastery

Monday

- Breakfast: Quinoa Fruit Salad
- Lunch: Quinoa Stuffed Bell Peppers
- Dinner: Grilled Chicken with Herb Salad

Tuesday

- Breakfast: Spelt Pancakes
- Lunch: Spicy Chickpea Stew
- Dinner: Turkey Meatballs in Tomato Sauce

Wednesday

- Breakfast: Chia Seed Pudding
- Lunch: Butternut Squash Soup
- Dinner: Beef Stir-Fry with Alkaline Vegetables

Thursday

- Breakfast: Buckwheat Porridge
- Lunch: Zucchini Noodles with Pesto
- Dinner: Lamb Chops with Mint Pesto

Friday

- Breakfast: Kamut Flour Waffles
- Lunch: Lentil and Vegetable Curry

- Dinner: Roasted Duck with Orange Glaze

Saturday

- Breakfast: Alkaline Avocado Bowl
- Lunch: Stuffed Portobello Mushrooms
- Dinner: Venison Stew with Root Vegetables

Sunday

- Breakfast: Millet and Cinnamon Apple Bowl
- Lunch: Wild Rice and Mushroom Pilaf
- Dinner: Pork Tenderloin with Apple Compote

Daily Snacks (Choose One):

- Almond Butter and Celery Sticks
- Kale Chips
- Cucumber and Hummus Bites
- Coconut Yogurt with Nuts and Seeds
- Fruit Leather with Alkaline Fruits
- Spiced Pumpkin Seeds
- Avocado and Tomato Salsa
- Raw Energy Balls
- Vegetable Spring Rolls
- Homemade Alkaline Crackers

Tips and Strategies for a Long, Healthy Life

While there is no one-size-fits-all solution to longevity, evidence suggests that adopting an alkaline lifestyle will help you live longer and healthier.

By focusing on nourishing your body with alkaline-forming foods and adopting healthy practices, you can lay the groundwork for bright well-being and potentially extend your life.

Here are some important guidelines and tactics for maximizing the alkaline advantage and promoting longevity:

- Prioritize alkaline-forming foods. Make fruits, vegetables, nuts, seeds, and legumes the highlight of your meal. These foods include critical nutrients, antioxidants, and minerals that help maintain a good pH balance and protect against chronic diseases.
- Limit Acid-Forming Foods: Reduce or eliminate processed foods, refined sugars, excess animal products, and unhealthy fats. These foods can upset your body's pH equilibrium, resulting in inflammation and other health difficulties.
- Hydrate wisely: Drink plenty of alkaline water throughout the day to flush out toxins and stay hydrated. For added flavour and health advantages, try herbal teas or infused water.
- Embrace Regular Exercise: Do moderate-intensity physical activity most days of the week. Exercise promotes a healthy weight, strengthens bones and muscles, improves cardiovascular health, and alleviates stress.

- Manage Stress: Chronic stress can have a negative impact on your health, leading to inflammation and a variety of ailments. Find healthy stress-management techniques, such as yoga, meditation, deep breathing exercises, or spending time outside.

- Prioritize Sleep: Aim for 7-8 hours of good sleep per night. Sleep is critical for cellular repair, hormone control, and overall health.

- Cultivate Social Connections: Research has linked strong social relationships to improved health and lifespan. Spend time with your loved ones, participate in social events, and form supportive relationships.

- Limit your intake of alcohol and caffeine, as both can disturb pH balance and cause dehydration. Consume them in moderation, or explore alternatives such as herbal teas and infused water.

- Practice Mindful Eating: Pay attention to your body's hunger and fullness signals. Eat gently, relish every bite, and avoid distractions while eating. This can help you avoid overeating and improve digestion.

- Regular Health Checkups: Make regular appointments with your doctor to monitor your health and treat any potential problems early on.

By adopting these techniques and strategies into your daily routine, you may establish a sustained alkaline lifestyle that nourishes your body, promotes longevity, and improves your overall well-being.

Remember that the goal is growth, not perfection. Even tiny modifications can have a significant impact over time.

Your Alkaline Shopping Plan and lists

Transforming your kitchen into an alkaline haven is simpler than you would believe! With a well-stocked pantry and refrigerator, you'll have everything you need to prepare tasty, pH-balancing meals that nourish both your body and your taste buds.

Shopping strategies:

- Shop the Perimeter: The exterior aisles of most grocery shops have fresh vegetables, dairy, and meat. Concentrate your purchasing in these areas, which contain the majority of alkaline-forming foods.
- Choose Organic When Possible: Organic fruit is grown without the use of synthetic pesticides and fertilizers, which can contribute to acidity. While organic options may be slightly more expensive, they can be beneficial to your health.
- Read labels carefully. Avoid manufactured foods with lengthy ingredient lists including fake additives, extra sugars, and harmful fats. Choose complete, unprocessed meals wherever possible.
- Buy in bulk: To save money and guarantee that you always have ingredients on hand, stock up on non-perishable alkaline staples such as nuts, seeds, and legumes.
- Plan Your Meals: Making a weekly food plan will help you remain on track and avoid impulse buying. Choose meals that include a variety of alkaline-forming foods to ensure you obtain a diverse spectrum of nutrients.

Alkaline Grocery Lists:

Produce:

- Leafy greens include kale, spinach, romaine lettuce, collard greens, and Swiss chard.
- Cruciferous vegetables include broccoli, cauliflower, Brussels sprouts, and cabbage.
- Root veggies include sweet potatoes, beets, carrots, and parsnips.
- Other veggies include cucumbers, bell peppers, celery, zucchini, asparagus, green beans, onions, garlic, and tomatoes.
- Fruits: lemons, limes, strawberries, avocados, melons, grapefruit.

Pantry staples:

- Nuts and seeds: almonds, cashews, walnuts, chia, flax, pumpkin, and hemp seeds.
- legumes: lentils, chickpeas, black beans, kidney beans.
- Healthy fats include olive oil, avocado oil, and coconut oil.
- herbs and spices: basil, parsley, cilantro, ginger, turmeric, and cinnamon.
- Other options include quinoa, millet, brown rice (in moderation), herbal teas, and alkaline water.

Refrigerator essentials:

- Plant-based milk substitutes include almond milk, coconut milk, and oat milk.
- Tempeh or tofu (as preferred).
- Hummus or other alkaline dips.
- Fresh herbs.

With a well-stocked kitchen and a little planning, you can easily prepare tasty and healthy alkaline meals that will benefit your health and well-being. Happy shopping!

CHAPTER 3: BREAKFAST RECIPES

Alkaline Green Smoothie.

Serving Size: One.

Prep time: 5 minutes.

Ingredients:

- One cup spinach leaf.
- One tiny ripe banana.
- One-half avocado
- 1/2 cup chopped cucumber.
- One tablespoon of chia seeds.
- One cup of alkaline or coconut water.
- Ice cubes (Optional)

Instructions:

- In a blender, mix spinach, banana, avocado, cucumber, and chia seeds.
- Add alkaline or coconut water.
- Blend on high until smooth. If you want your smoothie to be colder, add ice cubes.
- Serve immediately.

Nutrition Information: Calories: 300; fat: 15g; carbohydrates: 45g; protein: 5g.

Quinoa Fruit Salad.

Serving Size: two.

Prep time: 15 minutes.

Cook time: 20 minutes.

Ingredients:

- One cup quinoa.
- Two glasses of water.
- 1/2 cup sliced strawberries.
- One-half cup blueberries
- 1/2 cup raspberries.
- 1/4 cup slivered almonds.
- 1/4 cup fresh mint, chopped
- Juice from 1 lemon

Instructions:

- Rinse the quinoa under cold water.
- In a pot, bring quinoa and water to a boil. Reduce the heat, cover, and let simmer for 15 minutes.
- Remove from heat and cover for 5 minutes. Fluff with a fork and allow to cool.
- In a large bowl, combine the chilled quinoa, berries, almonds, and mint.
- Drizzle with lemon juice and mix lightly.
- Serve cold or room temperature.

Nutrition Information: Calories: 320; fat: 9g; carbohydrates: 53g; protein: 12g.

Spelt Pancake

Serving Size: four.

Prep time: 10 minutes.

Cook time: 15 minutes.

Ingredients:

- One cup spelt flour.
- One tablespoon of baking powder.
- 1/4 teaspoon sea salt.
- One cup of almond milk.
- 1 tablespoon melted coconut oil.
- One tablespoon maple syrup.
- 1 teaspoon of vanilla extract.

Instructions:

- In a bowl, combine the spelt flour, baking powder, and sea salt.
- In another bowl, combine almond milk, melted coconut oil, maple syrup, and vanilla extract.
- Add wet ingredients to dry ingredients and mix until just blended.
- Heat a nonstick pan over medium heat, then spoon 1/4 cup batter into each pancake.
- Cook until bubbles appear on the surface, then turn and finish until golden brown.
- Add more maple syrup if desired.

Nutrition Information: Calories: 200; fat: 5g; carbohydrates: 35g; protein: 6g.

Chia Seed Pudding.

Serving Size: two.

Preparation time is 5 minutes (including overnight soak).

Ingredients:

- 1/4 cup of chia seeds.
- One cup of almond milk.
- 1/2 teaspoon vanilla extract.
- One tablespoon maple syrup.
- Fresh berries for topping.

Instructions:

- In a bowl, blend the chia seeds, almond milk, vanilla essence, and maple syrup.
- Stir well and set aside for 5 minutes. Stir again to avoid clumping.
- Cover and refrigerate overnight.
- In the morning, mix it well and top with fresh berries.
- Serve cold.

Nutrition Information: Calories: 150; fat: 8g; carbohydrates: 17g; protein: 5g.

Buckwheat Porridge.

Serving Size: two.

Prep time: 5 minutes.

Cooking Time: 10 minutes.

Ingredients:

- One cup of buckwheat groats
- Two glasses of water.
- 1/4 teaspoon sea salt.
- 1/2 teaspoon cinnamon.
- One-quarter cup almond milk
- One tablespoon maple syrup.
- Fresh fruit as a topping

Instructions:

- Rinse the buckwheat groats with cold water.
- In a pot, cook the buckwheat, water, and sea salt until boiling.
- Reduce heat, cover, and let simmer for 10 minutes.
- Remove from heat and cover for 5 minutes.
- Stir in the cinnamon, almond milk, and maple syrup.
- Serve topped with fresh fruit.

Nutrition Information: Calories: 320; fat: 3g; carbohydrates: 68g; protein: 12g.

Kamut Flour Waffles.

Serving Size: two waffles.

Prep time: 10 minutes.

Cook for 5 minutes per waffle.

Ingredients:

- One cup Kamut flour.
- 1 teaspoon of aluminium-free baking powder
- 1/4 teaspoon sea salt.
- One cup of almond milk.
- One tablespoon of grapeseed oil.
- One tablespoon of agave syrup

Instructions:

- Preheat the waffle iron.
- In a bowl, combine the Kamut flour, baking powder, and sea salt.
- In another bowl, combine the almond milk, grapeseed oil, and agave syrup.
- Combine the wet and dry ingredients and stir until smooth.
- Pour the batter onto the waffle iron and cook according the manufacturer's directions.
- Serve hot with your preferred alkaline-friendly toppings.

Nutrition Information: Calories: 290; fat: 8g; carbohydrates: 50g; protein: 8g.

Alkaline Avocado Bowl

Serving Size: One bowl.

Prep time: 5 minutes.

Ingredients:

- One ripe avocado, halved and pitted
- Half-cup cooked quinoa
- 1/4 cucumber, diced.
- One tablespoon of hemp seeds
- Juice from 1/2 lemon.
- Add sea salt and cayenne pepper to taste.

Instructions:

- Scoop off some of the avocado flesh to make a bigger cavity.
- In a bowl, combine the quinoa, cucumber, hemp seeds, lemon juice, sea salt, and cayenne pepper.
- Fill avocado halves with quinoa mixture.
- Serve immediately.

Nutrition Information: Calories: 330; fat: 23g; carbohydrates: 29g; protein: 9g.

Millet and Cinnamon Apple Bowl.

Serving Size: One bowl.

Prep time: 5 minutes.

Cook time: 20 minutes.

Ingredients:

- 1/2 cup millet.
- One cup of water.
- 1 apple (cored and cut)
- 1/2 teaspoon cinnamon.
- One tablespoon of almond butter.
- One tablespoon of agave syrup

Instructions:

- Rinse the millet under cold water.
- In a pot, combine the millet and water. Bring to a boil, then reduce the heat and cover for 20 minutes.
- Once cooked, fluff the millet with a fork and allow it cool slightly.
- Mix in the diced apples, cinnamon, almond butter, and agave syrup.
- Serve warm.

Nutrition Information: Calories: 310; fat: 8g; carbohydrates: 55g; protein: 6g.

Amaranth Porridge with Berries

Serving Size: One bowl.

Prep time: 5 minutes.

Cook time: 20 minutes.

Ingredients:

- 1/2 cup amaranth.
- 1-1/2 cups water
- 1/2 cup mixed berries.
- One tablespoon of coconut flakes
- One tablespoon of agave syrup

Instructions:

- Rinse amaranth with cold water.
- In a pot, combine the amaranth and water. Bring to a boil, then reduce the heat and cover for 20 minutes.
- After cooking, let it rest for 5 minutes.
- Garnish with mixed berries, coconut flakes, and agave syrup.
- Serve warm.

Nutrition Information: Calories: 280; fat: 5g; carbohydrates: 55g; protein: 7g.

Teff Grain Breakfast Bowl.

Serving Size: One bowl.

Prep time: 5 minutes.

Cook time: 15 minutes.

Ingredients:

- 1/2 cup teff grain.
- Two glasses of water.
- 1/4 teaspoon sea salt.
- 1/2 banana, sliced
- 1 tablespoon of chopped walnuts
- One tablespoon of agave syrup

Instructions:

- Rinse the teff grain with cool water.
- In a pot, combine the teff, water, and sea salt. Bring to a boil, then reduce the heat and cover for 15 minutes.
- After cooking, let it rest for 5 minutes.
- Garnish with banana slices, walnuts, and agave syrup.
- Serve warm.

Nutrition Information: Calories: 300; fat: 6g; carbohydrates: 57g; protein: 10g.

CHAPTER 4: PLANT-BASED RECIPES

Kale And Avocado Salad.

Serving Size: two.

Prep time: 10 minutes.

Ingredients:

- 2 cups kale, de-stemmed and chopped
- One ripe avocado, chopped
- 1/2 cup cherry tomatoes, cut in half
- 1/4 cup thinly sliced red onion.
- 2 tablespoons pumpkin seeds.
- 2 tablespoons lemon juice.
- One tablespoon olive oil.
- Add sea salt and black pepper to taste.

Instructions:

- In a large mixing bowl, combine kale, lemon juice, olive oil, sea salt, and black pepper. Massage until soft.
- Combine avocado, cherry tomatoes, red onion, and pumpkin seeds in a bowl.
- Toss gently to blend.
- Serve immediately or allow the flavors to mingle.

Nutrition Information: 250 calories; 20g fat; 18g carbohydrates; 6g protein.

Quinoa-Stuffed Bell Peppers.

Serving Size: four.

Prep time: 15 minutes.

Cook for 30 minutes.

Ingredients:

- 4 bell peppers with tops removed and seeded
- 1 cup cooked quinoa.
- 1/2 cup washed and drained black beans.
- 1/2 cup of corn kernels.
- 1/2 cup of diced tomatoes.
- 1/4 cup coarsely chopped red onion.
- 1/4 cup chopped cilantro.
- 1 teaspoon cumin.
- One teaspoon of chili powder
- Add sea salt to taste.

Instructions:

- Preheat the oven to 375° F (190° C).
- In a bowl, combine the cooked quinoa, black beans, corn, tomatoes, red onion, cilantro, cumin, chili powder, and sea salt.
- Stuff each bell pepper with quinoa mixture.
- Arrange the filled peppers in a baking dish and cover with foil.
- Bake for 30 minutes, until the peppers are soft.
- Serve hot.

Nutrition Information: Calories: 220; fat: 2g; carbohydrates: 42g; protein: 8g.

<u>**Spicy Chickpea Stew.**</u>

Serving Size: four.

Prep time: 10 minutes.

Cook time: 25 minutes.

Ingredients:

- 2 cups cooked chickpeas.
- One tablespoon olive oil.
- 1 onion, diced
- 2 garlic cloves, minced
- One teaspoon turmeric
- 1 teaspoon cumin.
- 1/2 teaspoon cayenne pepper.
- One can (14 ounces) of diced tomatoes
- Two cups of veggie broth.
- Add sea salt to taste.
- Fresh cilantro to garnish.

Instructions:

- Heat the olive oil in a big pot over medium heat.
- Sauté the onion and garlic until transparent.
- Stir in the turmeric, cumin, and cayenne pepper for about 1 minute.
- Stir in the chickpeas, diced tomatoes, and vegetable broth.
- Bring to a boil, then reduce the heat and simmer for 20 minutes.
- Sprinkle with sea salt and sprinkle with cilantro before serving.

Nutrition Information: Calories: 260; fat: 6g; carbohydrates: 40g; protein: 12g.

Butternut Squash Soup.

Serving Size: four.

Prep time: 15 minutes.

Cook for 30 minutes.

Ingredients:

- 4 cups butternut squash, peeled and diced
- One tablespoon olive oil.
- 1 onion, diced
- 3 garlic cloves, minced
- Four cups of veggie broth.
- One teaspoon of cinnamon.
- 1/2 teaspoon nutmeg.
- Add sea salt and black pepper to taste.

Instructions:

- In a big pot, heat the olive oil over medium heat.
- Sauté onion and garlic till tender.
- Combine the butternut squash, vegetable broth, cinnamon, and nutmeg.
- Bring to a boil, then reduce heat and simmer for 25 minutes, or until the squash is soft.
- Using an immersion blender, purée the soup until smooth.
- Season with sea salt and black pepper.
- Serve hot.

Nutrition Information: Calories: 180; fat: 4g; carbohydrates: 37g; protein: 3g.

Zucchini Noodles with Pesto.

Serving Size: two.

Prep time: 15 minutes.

Ingredients:

- Two medium zucchinis, spiralized
- One cup fresh basil leaf.
- One-quarter cup pine nuts
- Two garlic cloves.
- One-quarter cup olive oil
- Juice from 1 lemon
- Add sea salt to taste.

Instructions:

- In a food processor, mix together basil, pine nuts, garlic, olive oil, lemon juice, and sea salt. To create pesto, blend until smooth.
- Toss spiralized zucchini with pesto until evenly covered.
- Serve immediately, with more pine nuts if preferred.

Nutrition Information: Calories: 290; fat: 26g; carbohydrates: 12g; protein: 4g.

Wild Rice and Mushroom Pilaf.

Serving Size: two.

Prep time: 10 minutes.

Cook for 45 minutes.

Ingredients:

- 1 cup washed wild rice.
- 2-1/2 cups vegetable broth
- One tablespoon olive oil.
- One small onion, chopped
- 2 cups sliced mushrooms.
- 2 garlic cloves, minced
- 1/4 teaspoon thyme.
- Add sea salt and black pepper to taste.

Instructions:

- In a saucepan, heat the wild rice and vegetable broth until boiling. Reduce the heat to low, cover, and simmer for 45 minutes.
- While the rice is cooking, heat the olive oil in a skillet over medium heat. Sauté the onion until transparent.
- Cook the mushrooms until they release moisture and begin to brown.
- Cook for a further minute after adding the garlic, thyme, sea salt, and black pepper.
- Once the rice is done, fluff it with a fork and stir in the mushroom mixture.
- Serve warm.

Nutrition Information: Calories 360; fat 7g; carbs 68g; protein 14g.

Lentils and Vegetable Curry

Serving Size: four.

Prep time: 15 minutes.

Cook for 30 minutes.

Ingredients:

- 1 cup washed green lentils.
- One tablespoon of coconut oil.
- 1 onion, chopped
- 2 garlic cloves, minced
- One tablespoon of curry powder
- 1 teaspoon cumin.
- 1/2 teaspoon turmeric.
- One can (14 ounces) of diced tomatoes
- Two cups of veggie broth.
- One cup cauliflower floret.
- 1 cup of chopped carrots.
- Add sea salt to taste.

Instructions:

- Heat the coconut oil in a big pot over medium heat. Add the onion and garlic and sauté until tender.
- Cook for 1 minute while stirring in the curry powder, cumin, and turmeric.
- Combine the lentils, diced tomatoes, vegetable broth, cauliflower, and carrots. Bring to a boil.
- Reduce the heat and simmer for 30 minutes, or until the lentils are cooked.
- Season with sea salt. Serve warm.

Nutrition Information: Calories: 280; fat: 4g; carbohydrates: 48g; protein: 16g.

Stuffed Portobello Mushroom

Serving Size: four.

Prep time: 15 minutes.

Cook time: 20 minutes.

Ingredients:

- 4 large portobello mushrooms with stems removed.
- One tablespoon olive oil.
- 1/2 cup cooked quinoa.
- 1/4 cup diced red bell pepper.
- 1/4 cup chopped zucchini.
- 2 tablespoons pine nuts.
- One tablespoon nutritional yeast.
- 1/4 teaspoon garlic powder.
- Add sea salt and black pepper to taste.

Instructions:

- Preheat the oven to 375° F (190° C).
- Brush the portobello caps with olive oil and set them on a baking sheet.
- In a bowl, mix cooked quinoa, bell pepper, zucchini, pine nuts, nutritional yeast, garlic powder, sea salt, and black pepper.
- Stuff each mushroom cap with quinoa mixture.
- Bake for 20 minutes, until the mushrooms are soft.
- Serve hot.

Nutrition Information: Calories: 200; fat: 9g; carbohydrates: 23g; protein: 9g.

Eggplant and Tomato Bake.

Serving Size: four.

Prep time: 15 minutes.

Cooking Time: 40 minutes.

Ingredients:

- 1 large eggplant, cut into half-inch rounds
- Two cups of diced tomatoes.
- 1 onion, sliced
- 3 garlic cloves, minced
- 1/4 cup of fresh basil, chopped
- 2 tablespoons olive oil.
- Add sea salt and black pepper to taste.

Instructions:

- Preheat the oven to 375° F (190° C).
- In a baking dish, arrange the eggplant, tomatoes, onion, and garlic.
- Drizzle with olive oil, then season with sea salt and black pepper.
- Cover with foil and bake for 30 minutes.
- Remove the foil, sprinkle with basil, and bake for another 10 minutes.
- Serve hot.

Nutrition Information: Calories: 130; fat: 7g; carbohydrates: 17g; protein: 3g.

<u>**Sweet Potato and Black Bean Chili.**</u>

Serving Size: four.

Prep time: 15 minutes.

Cook time: 35 minutes.

Ingredients:

- Two medium sweet potatoes, peeled and diced
- One tablespoon olive oil.
- 1 onion, diced
- 2 garlic cloves, minced
- 1 can (14 oz) washed and drained black beans.
- One can (14 ounces) of diced tomatoes
- Two cups of veggie broth.
- One tablespoon of chili powder
- 1 teaspoon cumin.
- Add sea salt to taste.

Instructions:

- Heat the olive oil in a big pot over medium heat. Add the onion and garlic and sauté until tender.
- Combine the sweet potatoes, black beans, diced tomatoes, vegetable broth, chili powder, and cumin.
- Bring to a boil, then reduce the heat and simmer for 30 minutes, or until the sweet potatoes are cooked.
- Season with sea salt. Serve warm.

Nutrition Information: Calories: 270; fat: 4g; carbohydrates: 51g; protein: 9g.

CHAPTER 5: SEAFOOD RECIPES

Grilled Lemon and Garlic Salmon

Serving Size: two.

Prep time: 10 minutes.

Cook time: 15 minutes.

Ingredients:

- Two salmon fillets, 6 ounces apiece.
- 2 tablespoons olive oil.
- 4 garlic cloves, minced
- 1 lemon (juice and zest)
- One teaspoon of sea salt.
- 1/2 teaspoon black pepper.
- Fresh dill as garnish

Instructions:

- Preheat the grill to medium-high heat.
- In a bowl, combine the olive oil, garlic, lemon juice and zest, salt, and pepper.
- Coat the salmon fillets in the mixture and marinate for 10 minutes.
- Grill the salmon, skin side down, for 7-8 minutes.
- Flip gently and grill for a further 7-8 minutes, or until desired doneness.
- Garnish with fresh dill and serve.

Nutrition Information: Calories: 367, protein: 34g, carbohydrates: 3g, fat: 24g.

Baked Sea Bass and Asparagus

Serving Size: two.

Prep time: 15 minutes.

Cook time: 20 minutes.

Ingredients:

- Two sea bass fillets (6 ounces each)
- 1 bunch asparagus, trimmed
- 2 tablespoons olive oil.
- One lemon, cut
- One teaspoon of sea salt.
- 1/2 teaspoon black pepper.

Instructions:

- Preheat the oven to 400°F (200° C).
- Place the asparagus on a baking sheet and drizzle with 1 tablespoon olive oil. Season with salt and pepper.
- Arrange sea bass fillets on top of asparagus.
- Drizzle the remaining olive oil over the sea bass, then top with lemon wedges.
- Bake for 20 minutes, or until the fish flakes easily with a fork.
- Serve immediately.

Nutrition Information: Calories: 295, protein: 23g, carbohydrates: 4g, fat: 21g.

Shrimp & Arugula Salad

Serving Size: four.

Prep time: 15 minutes.

Cook for 5 minutes.

Ingredients:

- 1 pound of shrimp, peeled and deveined
- Four cups arugula.
- One avocado, sliced
- One-quarter cup pine nuts
- 2 tablespoons olive oil.
- 1 lemon (juice and zest)
- One teaspoon of sea salt.
- 1/2 teaspoon black pepper.

Instructions:

- Heat 1 tbsp olive oil in a pan on medium heat.
- Season the shrimp with salt and pepper, then cook for 2-3 minutes on each side.
- In a large mixing basin, combine arugula, avocado, and pine nuts.
- Mix cooked shrimp into the salad.
- Drizzle with lemon juice, zest, and the remaining olive oil.
- Toss lightly, then serve.

Nutrition Information: Calories: 242; protein: 25g; carbohydrates: 6g; fat: 14g.

Herb-Crusted Cod

Serving Size: two.

Prep time: 10 minutes.

Cook time: 15 minutes.

Ingredients:

- Two cod fillets, 6 ounces apiece.
- One-quarter cup almond flour
- Two tablespoons of mixed herbs (parsley, thyme, basil)
- 2 tablespoons olive oil.
- 1 lemon (juice and zest)
- One teaspoon of sea salt.
- 1/2 teaspoon black pepper.

Instructions:

- Preheat the oven to 400°F (200° C).
- Combine almond flour, herbs, salt, and pepper in a bowl.
- Coat the cod fillets in olive oil and press them into the herb mixture.
- Place on a prepared baking sheet and bake for 15 minutes, or until golden and flaky.
- Drizzle with lemon juice and zest before serving.

Nutrition Information: Calories: 280, protein: 28g, carbohydrates: 4g, fat: 17g.

Seafood Quinoa Paella.

Serving Size: four.

Prep time: 20 minutes.

Cook for 30 minutes.

Ingredients:

- 1 cup washed quinoa.
- Two cups of veggie broth.
- 1-pound mixed seafood (shrimp, scallops, and mussels)
- One red bell pepper, sliced
- 1/2 cup peas.
- 1/4 cup chopped parsley.
- 2 tablespoons olive oil.
- One teaspoon turmeric
- One teaspoon of sea salt.
- 1/2 teaspoon black pepper.

Instructions:

- In a large pan, heat the olive oil over medium heat.
- Add the quinoa and toast for 2 minutes.
- Combine the vegetable broth, turmeric, salt, and pepper. Bring to a boil.
- Reduce heat, cover, and let simmer for 15 minutes.
- Stir in the shrimp, bell peppers, and peas. Cook for an additional ten minutes.
- Garnish with parsley and serve.

Nutrition Information: Calories: 345, protein: 29g, carbohydrates: 33g, fat: 10g.

Alkaline Fish Tacos.

Serving Size: two.

Prep time: 15 minutes.

Cooking Time: 10 minutes.

Ingredients:

- 2 white fish fillets, 6 oz each.
- One tablespoon olive oil.
- 1 teaspoon cumin.
- 1/2 teaspoon paprika.
- 1/4 teaspoon sea salt.
- Four corn tortillas.
- One cup of shredded lettuce.
- One avocado, sliced
- 1/2 cup of diced tomatoes.
- 1/4 cup of chopped cilantro.

Instructions:

- Preheat the grill to medium.
- Combine olive oil, cumin, paprika, and sea salt in a bowl.
- Coat the fish fillets in the spice mixture.
- Grill fish for 5 minutes per side.
- Grill tortillas for 1 minute per side.
- Make tacos using lettuce, fish, avocado, tomatoes, and cilantro.

Nutrition Information: Calories: 390, protein: 28g, carbohydrates: 30g, fat: 18g.

<u>**Mussels In Tomato Broth.**</u>

Serving Size: four.

Prep time: 10 minutes.

Cook time: 15 minutes.

Ingredients:

- 2 pounds of mussels, cleaned
- One tablespoon olive oil.
- 4 garlic cloves, minced
- One cup of diced tomatoes.
- One-half cup vegetable broth
- 1/4 cup of minced parsley.
- One lemon, juice only.
- 1/4 teaspoon sea salt.

Instructions:

- Heat the olive oil in a pot over medium heat.
- Add the garlic and sauté until fragrant.
- Add the tomatoes and broth, and bring to a boil.
- Add the mussels, cover, and cook until they open.
- Discard any unopened mussels.
- Before serving, stir in the parsley and lemon juice.

Nutrition Information: Calories: 175. Protein: 22g. Carbs: 9g. Fat: 6g.

Scallops and Zesty Quinoa

Serving Size: two.

Prep time: 20 minutes.

Cook time: 15 minutes.

Ingredients:

- 1/2 cup quinoa.
- One cup of water.
- One tablespoon olive oil.
- Six big scallops.
- 1/2 teaspoon grated lemon zest.
- 1/4 cup of chopped mint.
- 1/4 teaspoon sea salt.

Instructions:

- Rinse quinoa and cook it in water according to package directions.
- Heat the olive oil in a pan over medium-high heat.
- Season the scallops with salt and sear until brown.
- Fluff the quinoa with a fork, then whisk in the lemon zest and mint.
- Serve scallops with quinoa.

Nutrition Information: Calories: 320, protein: 20g, carbohydrates: 35g, fat: 10g.

Tuna & Avocado Poke Bowl

Serving Size: two.

Prep time: 20 minutes.

Ingredients:

- 1/2-pound sushi-grade tuna, cubed
- One avocado, diced
- One cup of cooked brown rice.
- 1/2 cup of diced cucumber.
- 2 tbsp soy sauce (alkaline friendly)
- One tablespoon of sesame oil.
- One teaspoon of sesame seeds
- 1/4 cup of sliced green onions.

Instructions:

- Put brown rice in two bowls.
- Garnish with tuna, avocado, and cucumber.
- Combine soy sauce and sesame oil; drizzle over bowls.
- Garnish with sesame seeds and green onions.

Nutrition Information: Calories: 480, protein: 28g, carbohydrates: 38g, fat: 24g.

Sardine and Spinach Salad.

Serving Size: two.

Prep time: 10 minutes.

Ingredients:

- Four cups of baby spinach
- 1 can sardines in olive oil, drained
- 1/2 avocado, sliced
- 1/4 cup of sliced red onion.
- 1/2 lemon, juice only.
- One tablespoon olive oil.
- 1/4 teaspoon sea salt.

Instructions:

- Arrange the spinach on plates.
- Garnish with sardines, avocado, and red onion.
- Whisk together the lemon juice, olive oil, and salt.
- Drizzle dressing over salad.

Nutrition Information: Calories: 310, protein: 23g, carbohydrates: 8g, fat: 22g.

CHAPTER 6: MEAT RECIPES

Grilled Chicken and Herb Salad.

Serving Size: two.

Prep time: 15 minutes.

Cook time: 20 minutes.

Ingredients:

- Two chicken breasts, 6 ounces each.
- One tablespoon olive oil.
- One teaspoon of dried oregano.
- One teaspoon dried thyme.
- One teaspoon of dried rosemary
- 1/2 teaspoon black pepper.
- 1/2 teaspoon sea salt.
- 4 cups mixed greens (kale, spinach, and arugula).
- 1/4 cup fresh parsley, chopped
- 1/4 cup of fresh basil, chopped
- 2 tablespoons lemon juice.

Instructions:

- Preheat the grill to medium-high heat.
- Coat chicken in olive oil and season with herbs, salt, and pepper.
- Grill chicken for 10 minutes per side.
- Combine mixed greens, parsley, basil, and lemon juice.
- Place grilled chicken on top of the herb salad.

Nutrition Information: 320 calories, 35g protein, 4g carbs, and 18g fat.

Turkey Meatballs with Tomato Sauce.

Serving Size: four.

Prep time: 20 minutes.

Cook for 30 minutes.

Ingredients:

- One pound of ground turkey
- 1 egg
- One-half cup almond flour
- 1/4 cup fresh parsley, chopped
- One teaspoon of sea salt.
- 1/2 teaspoon black pepper.
- 2 cups tomato sauce, alkaline-friendly.

Instructions:

- Preheat the oven to 375° F (190° C).
- Combine the ground turkey, egg, almond flour, parsley, salt, and pepper.
- Roll into 1-inch meatballs and lay them on a baking pan.
- Bake for twenty minutes.
- Heat tomato sauce in a pan, then add meatballs. Simmer for ten minutes.
- Serve hot.

Nutrition Information: Calories: 250, protein: 28g, carbohydrates: 8g, fat: 12g.

Beef Stir-Fry with Alkaline Vegetables.

Serving Size: two.

Prep time: 15 minutes.

Cooking Time: 10 minutes.

Ingredients:

- 1/2-pound beef strips
- One tablespoon of coconut oil.
- Two cups of mixed alkaline vegetables (broccoli, bell peppers, zucchini)
- 1 tablespoon of tamari sauce (alkaline-friendly)
- 1 tsp grated ginger.
- One garlic clove, minced
- 1/2 teaspoon sea salt.

Instructions:

- Cook coconut oil in a wok over high heat.
- Stir-fry the beef strips for three minutes.
- Combine the vegetables, tamari, ginger, and garlic. Stir fry for an additional 7 minutes.
- Sprinkle with sea salt and serve immediately.

Nutrition Information: Calories: 300, protein: 25g, carbohydrates: 10g, fat: 18g.

Lamb Chops with Mint Pesto.

Serving Size: two.

Prep time: 10 minutes.

Cook time: 14 minutes.

Ingredients:

- Four lamb chops.
- One tablespoon olive oil.
- 1/2 teaspoon sea salt.
- One-quarter teaspoon black pepper
- One cup of fresh mint leaves
- 1/4 cup olive oil for pesto.
- One-quarter cup almonds
- One garlic clove.
- One tablespoon of lemon juice.

Instructions:

- Preheat the grill to medium heat.
- Season the lamb chops with olive oil, salt, and pepper.
- Grill for 7 minutes per side.
- To make the pesto, combine mint, olive oil, almonds, garlic, and lemon juice until smooth.
- Serve lamb chops with a dollop of mint pesto.

Nutrition Information: Calories: 450, protein: 38g, carbohydrates: 2g, fat: 32g.

Roasted Duck with Orange Glaze.

Serving Size: four.

Prep time: 20 minutes.

Cooking Time: 2 hours.

Ingredients:

- One whole duck (5 pounds)
- 1 orange quartered
- One teaspoon of sea salt.
- 1/2 teaspoon black pepper.
- 1/2 cup of orange juice.
- 1 tablespoon honey.
- 1 teaspoon of apple cider vinegar.

Instructions:

- Preheat the oven to 350°F (175° C).
- Season duck with salt and pepper, then fill with orange quarters.
- Roast for an hour and forty minutes.
- For the glaze, combine orange juice, honey, and vinegar. Brush over the duck.
- Roast for a further 20 minutes, or until golden.

Nutrition Information: Calories: 560, protein: 52g, carbohydrates: 12g, fat: 34g.

Venison Stew with Root Vegetables

Serving Size: four.

Prep time: 20 minutes.

Cooking Time: 2 hours.

Ingredients:

- 1 pound venison, diced
- Two cups of alkaline vegetable broth.
- 1 cup turnips, diced
- 1 cup parsnips, diced
- 1 cup chopped carrots.
- 1 onion, diced
- 2 garlic cloves, minced
- One tablespoon olive oil.
- 1 teaspoon thyme.
- One bay leaf.
- Add sea salt and black pepper to taste.

Instructions:

- In a big pot, heat the olive oil over medium heat.
- Add the venison and sear until browned.
- Add the garlic and onion and sauté until transparent.
- Pour in the vegetable broth and add the root vegetables, thyme, and bay leaf.
- Bring to a boil, then reduce to a low heat and simmer for two hours.
- Add sea salt and black pepper to taste.

Nutrition Information: Calories: 300, protein: 35g, carbohydrates: 20g, fat: 8g.

Pork Tenderloin with Apple Compote

Serving Size: four.

Prep time: 15 minutes.

Cook time: 25 minutes.

Ingredients:

- 1 pound pork tenderloin.
- Two apples, peeled and diced
- One tablespoon olive oil.
- 1/4 cup thinly sliced red onion.
- One teaspoon Dijon mustard
- 1/4 teaspoon cinnamon.
- Add sea salt and black pepper to taste.

Instructions:

- Preheat the oven to 375° F (190° C).
- Season the pork with salt, pepper, and cinnamon.
- Heat olive oil in a skillet, then brown the pork on all sides.
- Place pork in the oven and cook for 20 minutes.
- Sauté the apples and onion in the same skillet until tender.
- Stir in the Dijon mustard and simmer for another 5 minutes.
- Slice the pork and serve with apple compote.

Nutrition Information: 240 calories, 24g protein, 15g carbs, and 9g fat.

Buffalo Cauliflower Bites.

Serving Size: four.

Prep time: 10 minutes.

Cook time: 20 minutes.

Ingredients:

- Cut 1 head of cauliflower into florets.
- One-half cup almond flour
- One-half cup water
- One teaspoon garlic powder.
- 1/2 cup spicy sauce (alkaline friendly)
- One tablespoon olive oil.

Instructions:

- Preheat the oven to 450°F (230° C).
- Combine almond flour, water, and garlic powder to form a batter.
- Dip cauliflower florets into batter and lay on a baking pan.
- Drizzle with olive oil and bake 20 minutes.
- Toss cooked cauliflower with hot sauce and serve.

Nutrition Information: 150 calories, 5g protein, 18g carbs, and 7g fat.

Chicken Avocado Lettuce Wraps.

Serving Size: four.

Prep time: 10 minutes.

Ingredients:

- 2 cups of cooked chicken, shredded
- Two avocados, mashed
- 1/4 cup coarsely chopped red onion.
- 1 tablespoon of lime juice.
- 1/4 cup chopped cilantro.
- Eight lettuce leaves.
- Add sea salt and black pepper to taste.

Instructions:

- In a bowl, combine the chicken, avocado, onion, lime juice, and cilantro.
- Season with salt and pepper.
- Spoon the mixture into the lettuce leaves and fold to wrap.

Nutrition Information: 220 calories, 14g protein, 8g carbs, and 16g fat.

Bison Burgers with Alkaline Slaw

Serving Size: four.

Prep time: 15 minutes.

Cooking Time: 10 minutes.

Ingredients:

- One pound ground bison.
- 1/4 cup shredded red cabbage.
- 1/4 cup shredded carrot.
- 1/4 cup of apple cider vinegar.
- One tablespoon olive oil.
- Four whole grain buns.
- Add sea salt and black pepper to taste.

Instructions:

- Form four bison patties and season with salt and pepper.
- Heat a grill pan over medium heat, then cook patties for 5 minutes on each side.
- To make the slaw, combine cabbage, carrots, and vinegar.
- Serve burgers on buns topped with alkaline slaw.

Nutrition Information: Calories: 320, protein: 26g, carbohydrates: 22g, fat: 14g.

CHAPTER 7: SNACKS RECIPES

Almond Butter with Celery Sticks

Serving Size: two.

Prep time: 10 minutes.

Ingredients:

- Four huge celery sticks.
- Four tablespoons almond butter.

Instructions:

- Wash and dry the celery sticks.
- Cut them into 3-inch pieces.
- Place 1 tablespoon almond butter in the groove of each celery stick.

Nutrition Information: Calories: 98, protein: 2g, carbohydrates: 3g, fat: 9g.

Kale Chips.

Serving Size: two.

Prep time: 5 minutes.

Cooking Time: 10 minutes.

Ingredients:

- 1 bunch of kale with stems removed.
- One tablespoon olive oil.
- One pinch of sea salt.

Instructions:

- Preheat the oven to 350°F (175° C).
- Tear the kale into bite-size pieces.
- Toss in olive oil and sea salt.
- Spread on a baking sheet and bake until the edges are crispy, about 10 minutes.

Nutrition Information: 110 calories, 3g protein, 10g carbs, and 7g fat.

Cucumber and Hummus Bites.

Serving Size: four.

Prep time: 10 minutes.

Ingredients:

- 1 large cucumber sliced into rounds.
- One cup hummus.
- Paprika for garnish.

Instructions:

- Place cucumber rounds on a plate.
- Top each with a scoop of hummus.
- Season with paprika and serve.

Nutrition Information: Calories: 60, protein: 3g, carbohydrates: 5g, fat: 4g.

Coconut Yogurt with Nuts and Seeds

Serving Size: two.

Prep time: 5 minutes.

Ingredients:

- One cup of coconut yogurt.
- 1 tbsp chopped almonds.
- One tablespoon of pumpkin seeds
- One tablespoon of sunflower seeds

Instructions:

- Spoon coconut yogurt into bowls.
- Garnish with almonds, pumpkin seeds, and sunflower seeds.

Nutrition Information: 180 calories, 4g protein, 7g carbohydrates, and 15g fat.

Fruit Leather with Alkaline Fruits.

Serving Size: 10 strips.

Prep time: 15 minutes.

Cook time: three hours.

Ingredients:

- 2 cups of mixed alkaline fruits (berries, kiwi, and apples).
- One-quarter cup water
- One tablespoon of lemon juice.

Instructions:

- Preheat the oven to 170°F (75° C).
- Puree the fruits with water and lemon juice until smooth.
- Place a silicone baking mat on a baking sheet and spread the puree evenly.
- Dry in the oven for approximately 3 hours, until sticky.
- Once cool, cut into strips.

Nutrition Information: Calories: 45 per strip; protein: 0.5g; carbohydrates: 10g; fat: 0.2g.

Spiced Pumpkin Seeds.

Serving Size: four.

Prep time: 10 minutes.

Cook time: 15 minutes.

Ingredients:

- One cup pumpkin seed.
- One tablespoon olive oil.
- 1/2 teaspoon sea salt.
- 1/4 teaspoon cayenne pepper.
- 1/4 teaspoon garlic powder.

Instructions:

- Preheat the oven to 350°F (175° C).
- Combine pumpkin seeds, olive oil, sea salt, cayenne pepper, and garlic powder.
- Spread evenly across a baking sheet.
- Bake for 15 minutes, until brown and crispy.

Nutrition Information: 180 calories, 9g protein, 3g carbohydrates, and 15g fat.

Avocado & Tomato Salsa

Serving Size: four.

Prep time: 10 minutes.

Ingredients:

- Two ripe avocados, chopped
- 1 cup chopped tomatoes.
- 1/4 cup coarsely chopped red onion.
- 1/4 cup freshly minced cilantro.
- 2 tablespoons lime juice.
- Add sea salt and black pepper to taste.

Instructions:

- In a bowl, combine avocados, tomatoes, onion, and cilantro.
- Drizzle with lime juice, then season with salt and pepper.
- Gently mix and serve.

Nutrition Information: Calories: 160, protein: 2g, carbohydrates: 9g, fat: 14g.

Raw Energy Balls.

Serving Size: twelve balls.

Prep time: 15 minutes.

Ingredients:

- One cup raw almond.
- 1/2 cup of raw walnuts.
- 1 cup of pitted dates
- 2 tablespoons raw cacao powder.
- 1/4 teaspoon sea salt.
- 1–2 tablespoons water

Instructions:

- Using a food processor, combine almonds and walnuts until crumbly.
- Combine the dates, cacao powder, and sea salt. Process until sticky.
- Add water as needed to make dough.
- Shape into balls and chill until set.

Nutrition Information: 120 calories, 3g protein, 14g carbs, and 7g fat.

Vegetable Spring Rolls.

Serving Size: 10 rolls.

Prep time: 30 minutes.

Ingredients:

- Ten rice paper wraps.
- One cup of shredded cabbage.
- One cup julienned carrot.
- Half-cup finely sliced bell peppers
- 1/2 cup julienned cucumber.
- 1/4 cup of fresh basil leaves.
- 1/4 cup of fresh mint leaves.

Instructions:

- Soak rice paper wrappers in warm water until soft.
- Lay flat and arrange a small bit of each veggie in the center.
- Add basil and mint, then roll tightly and tuck in the sides.
- Serve with a dipping sauce.

Nutrition Information: Calories: 60; protein: 1g; carbohydrates: 14g; fat: 0g.

Homemade Alkaline Crackers.

Serving Size: 12 crackers.

Prep time: 10 minutes.

Cook for 30 minutes.

Ingredients:

- 1/2 cup chia seeds.
- One-half cup sesame seeds
- 1/2 cup pumpkin seeds.
- One-half cup sunflower seeds
- 1 garlic clove, crushed
- 1/2 teaspoon cayenne pepper.
- Add sea salt to taste.
- 1 1/4 cup water.

Instructions:

- Preheat the oven to 300°F (150° C).
- Mix together the seeds, garlic, cayenne pepper, salt, and water.
- Allow to sit for 10 minutes till the chia absorbs water.
- Spread the mixture onto a baking sheet lined with parchment paper.
- Bake for 30 minutes and turn halfway through.

Nutrition Information: 150 calories, 5g protein, 8g carbohydrates, and 11g fat.

CHAPTER 8: CREATING AN ALKALINE KITCHEN

Meal Planning and Prep

- Set Your Goals: Before you begin preparing, decide what your alkaline eating goals will be. Do you want to boost your energy, lose weight, or just feel better in general? Setting clear goals will allow you to personalise your diet plan to your individual requirements.

- Choose Your dishes: Choose dishes that include a variety of alkaline-forming foods, such as vegetables, fruits, nuts, seeds, and legumes. To keep your meals interesting and fulfilling, aim for a good balance of flavours and textures. Consider recipes that are easily adaptable for leftovers or batch cooking.

- Make a Weekly Meal Plan: Plan out your breakfast, lunch, dinner, and snacks for the week. Consider your schedule and preferences, and include a variety of recipes to prevent boredom.

Q: What is an alkaline diet?

A: The alkaline diet, also known as the acid-alkaline diet or alkaline ash diet, is based on the theory that the things we eat can influence our body's pH balance.

It emphasises eating alkaline-forming foods such fruits, vegetables, nuts, seeds, and legumes while avoiding acid-forming meals like processed foods, refined sweets, and excessive animal products.

Q: What are the advantages of an alkaline diet?

A: Proponents of the alkaline diet claim that it can provide a variety of health benefits, such as increased energy, weight loss, improved digestion, stronger bones, reduced inflammation, improved immune function, and clear skin.

Q: Does the alkaline diet actually change your body's pH?

A: While the things you eat can change the pH of your urine, they have little effect on your blood pH, which is carefully controlled by your body. An alkaline diet, on the other hand, can improve general health by emphasising nutrient-dense, complete foods.

Q: Is an alkaline diet safe?

A: Most people can safely consume an alkaline diet consisting of complete, unprocessed foods. However, before making significant dietary changes, you should consult with your doctor or a registered dietitian, especially if you have any underlying health conditions.

Q: Can I still consume meat on an alkaline diet?

A: While animal products are typically considered acid-forming, some people consume modest amounts of meat, fowl, or fish in moderation as part of an alkaline diet. If you decide to incorporate animal products, pick organic and grass-fed ones.

Q: Can I lose weight with an alkaline diet?

A: Many people lose weight on an alkaline diet because it emphasises whole, unprocessed foods and eliminates processed foods and refined sugars, which are high in calories and low in nutrients.

Q: Where do I find alkaline foods?

A: Most grocery stores have a large selection of alkaline-forming foods. Concentrate on the produce section for fresh fruits and veggies, the bulk section for nuts, seeds, and legumes, and the natural foods section for alkaline snacks and pantry staples.

Q: How long will it take to notice results from an alkaline diet?

A: The time it takes to see results varies according to individual characteristics and goals. Some people may notice an improvement in their energy levels and digestion after a few days, while others may take longer to see substantial results.

Q: Is the alkaline diet sustainable in the long run?

A: Over time, an alkaline diet can be a sustainable and enjoyable way to eat. By eating complete, unprocessed foods, you may nourish your body, improve health, and avoid chronic diseases.

CONCLUSION

Congratulations! You've completed this beginner's guide to alkaline eating, and I hope you feel empowered and encouraged to embark on this transforming journey. As you apply these principles and recipes to your life, keep in mind that every small step counts. Each alkalizing meal is an investment in your health, a foundation for a brighter, more vibrant future.

The alkaline lifestyle is not a fast fix; it is a lifetime commitment to supporting your body and respecting its inherent wisdom. By eating healthy meals, cultivating balance, and practicing mindfulness, you may create a ripple effect that spreads far beyond your plate. You're creating a healthy relationship with food, developing a stronger connection with your body, and laying the groundwork for long-term well-being.

As you continue on your alkaline journey, I encourage you to listen to your body, try different recipes, and discover the rhythm that works best for you. Remember, there is no one-size-fits-all solution. Allow oneself the flexibility to explore, adapt, and personalize this lifestyle.

And if you found this cookbook useful and educational, I'd appreciate your honest feedback. Your positive words can help spread the message of alkaline eating and inspire others to take control of their health.

Remember, this is just the beginning. The path to vibrant health is an ongoing exploration, and I am delighted to be a part of it.